The Best Soup Diet
Negative Calories Soup Diet

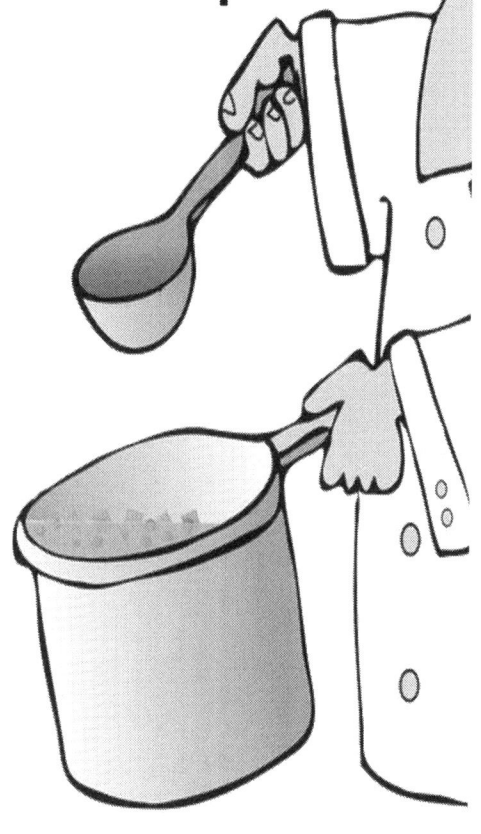

Norma Picon

The Best Soup Diet
Negative Calories Soup Diet

all rights reserved
Copyright © 2011 by Norma Picón
No part of this book may be used or reproduced in any manner whatsoever without written permission of the author or publisher.

Published in U.S.A.

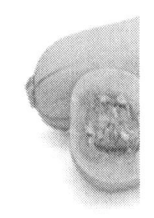

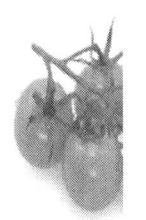

The Best Soup Diet
Negative Calories Soup Diet

ISBN-13:
978-1461109907

ISBN-10:
1461109906

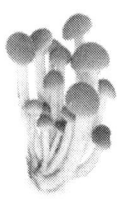

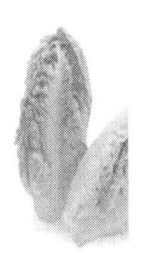

Note: the information in this book is true and correct to best of the author's knowledge. All recommendations are made as suggestions based on personal experience and without guarantees on the part of the author. The author disclaims all liability in connection with the use of this information.

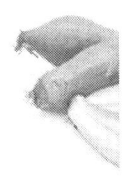

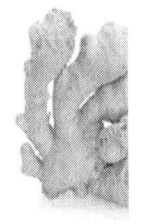

NorLu Creations
NorLu.com

Table of Contents

Dedication..IV

Introduction:
The Soup Diet Explained................... 5
What to buy.. 6
Benefits of Ingredients...................... 8

10 Days Planned Meals:
Day 1 & 2......................... 12
Day 3 & 4......................... 13
Day 5 & 6......................... 14
Day 7 & 8......................... 15
Day 9 & 10....................... 16

Recipes:
Soups.. 17

Salads... 29

Vegetables.. 41

Drinks & Desserts........................... 51

Other Detox diets defined:
Which Diet is Yours......................... 59
Boost Your Metabolic Rate.............. 61

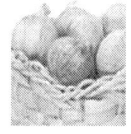

Weight Calendar......................... 62

Index... 64

Dedication

To my son Omar who is now my angel in heaven and is keeping an "eye" on his mommy. Thank you baby for loving my cooking.

to my sister, Dawn Marie who is my angel on earth

to all of you that are honoring yourselves by following a healthy diet

The supreme happiness of life is the conviction of being loved for yourself.
- Victor Hugo -

The Skinny Soup Diet Explained

The Cabbage Soup Diet came into popularity back in the 1980's more as a fad diet to lose weight fast, usually at a rate of 10 pounds a week, with the theory that the more of the soup that you eat, the more calories you will burn. As of today, no one has claimed credit for starting this diet. Many version of the Cabbage Diet are found on the internet, but the idea here is to offer an explanation as to why our version of the Soup Dieting works, and the different options you have to follow this diet successfully.

The talk now is about "negative calorie foods" we all know that all foods have calories, so what does this really mean? Simply, that there are certain foods which our body uses more calories to digest than the calories contained in the food; meaning, that the digestive system has to work harder in order to absorb the calories from these foods, turning them into fat-burning foods, thus the term "negative calorie foods"

Negative calorie foods contain enough vitamins and minerals to provide for enzyme production in sufficient quantities to break down its own calorie content, to convert these calories into energy, but additional calories

Soup Dieting will not only give you delicious soup recipes based on the concept of "negative calories foods" but will offer planned meals for 10 days, and explain the benefits of the main ingredients and foods.

Could you literally eat your way out to a slimmer and healthier you? Yes, you can...

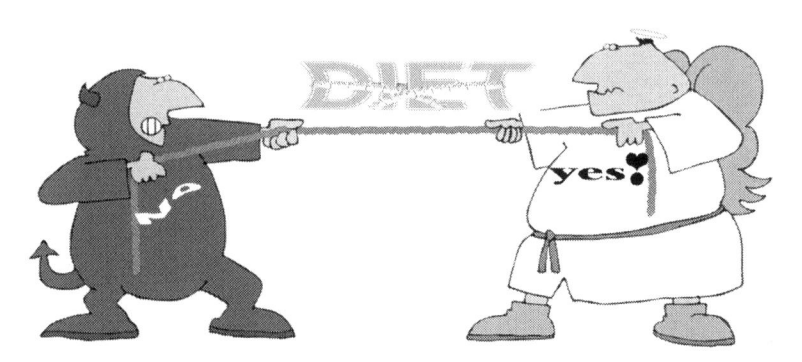

Grocery List

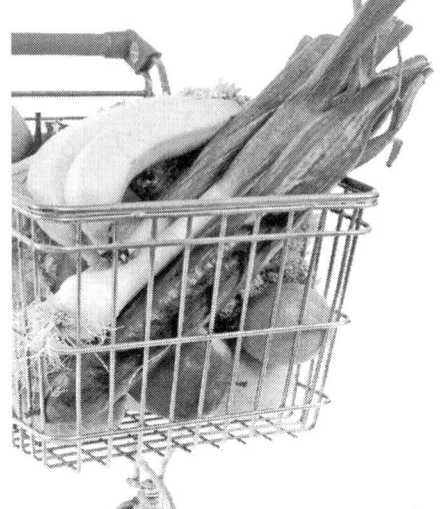

For your soup recipes:
- Broccoli
- Beets
- Green Cabbage
- Carrot
- Cauliflower
- Celery
- Chili Peppers
- Green Beans
- Zucchini
- Tomatoes

Flavoring for your soups and salads:

Fresh:
- Onions
- Garlic
- Parsley
- Cilantro
- Scallions
- Mint

Spices:
- Cayenne
- Cumin
- Sea Salt
- Black Pepper
- Oregano
- Apple Vinegar
- Virgin Olive Oil

Pantry Items:
- Canned diced tomatoes
- Tomato paste
- Canned Chickpeas
- Canned Cannelline Beans

Dessert items:
- Plain Greek yogurt
- Agave, organic

Grocery List

Negative Calorie List of Fruits & Vegetables

Fruits:
- Blueberry
- *Cranberry*
- *Grape Fruit*
- Mango
- Oranges
- *Pineapple*
- *Papaya*
- Raspberries
- Strawberries
- *Watermelon*

Salad Vegetables
- *Asparagus*
- Beets
- Broccoli
- Cauliflower
- Celery
- Cucumber
- Endive
- String Beans
- Lettuce
- Radishes
- Spinach

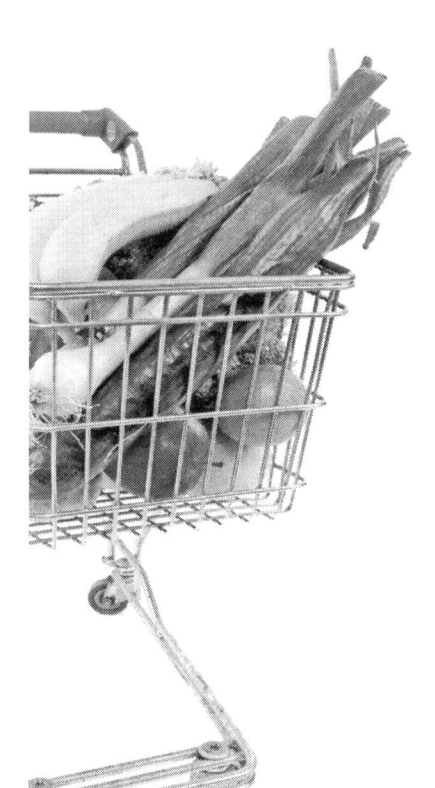

Following are foods which are consider "high in negative calories"

- Cranberry
- Grape Fruit
- Papaya
- Pineapple
- Watermelon
- Asparagus

Benefits of Ingredients

Green Vegetables: Dark leafy green vegetables are one of the best sources of nutrition, containing minerals including iron, calcium, potassium, and magnesium as well as vitamin K, C, E, and many of the B vitamins. Vitamin K alone can help regulate blood clotting and may help prevent and reduce inflammation, protecting us from inflammatory diseases including arthritis. Vegetables are naturally low in carbohydrates and rich in fiber, making them slow to digest, so you'll feel full longer.

Cabbage: Clinical research has revealed that cabbage is rich in antioxidants, high in Vitamin C, K, E, A, and B vitamins. Cabbage also provides an excellent source of dietary fiber; a combination that signals our genes to increase production of enzymes that activate the process of detoxification in our system, eliminating harmful compounds from our bodies. Not only is cabbage packed with health benefits, but one cup of cabbage soup has only 20-45 calories, depending in other products we may add.

Note: Knowing all the benefits of cabbage is important, but please keep in mind that cabbabe is high in Vitamin K, and if you are taking prescribed anticoagulants , cabbage is not recommended. The same care should be taken if you suffer from low thyroid hormone, as cabbage may interfere with the production of thyroid hormone. Please consult your medical provider.

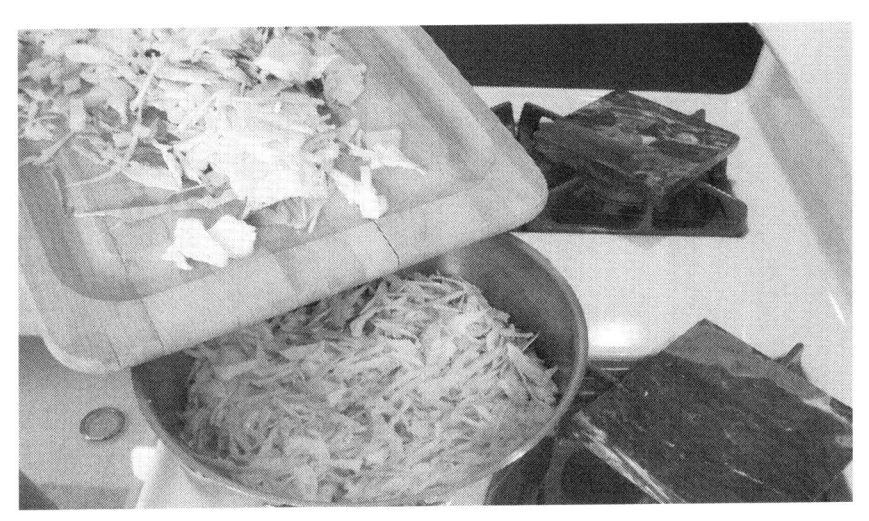

Benefits of Ingredients

Inulin: In the "Grocery List" you find Artichokes, Broccoli, Celery, Onions, Garlic, Asparagus, Leeks, Bananas, and a special section for Agave; all these foods are high in Inulin. Inulin is a naturally occurring plant fiber, which scientific studies have shown to help in weight loss, not only because it creates a sensation of fullness; but it cuts your craving for foods. Inulin is not digested or absorbed in the stomach, it goes directly to the bowel, where is turned into the kind of bacteria that improves bowel function and decreases the ability of the body to absorb fats.

Fruits: Those who eat generous amounts of fruits, are likely to have reduced risk of chronic diseases. Fruits contain essential vitamins, minerals, and fiber, and should be considered as a weight loss strategy by substituting fruits for higher calorie snack foods. Of special importance to incorporate in our Skinny Soup Diet are: Bananas, Grape Fruit, Papaya, Pineapple, Watermelon and Cranberry

Garlic: Studies have shown that garlic improves immune function, giving our natural defense system a boost, and helping it conserve our levels of antioxidants in our system. It is this strengthening of the immune system that aids in its support for other health related conditions. Studies have also shown that garlic has the ability to reduce the formation of cancerous cells, by blocking cancer causing compounds from forming, and slow the growth of tumor cells. Garlic helps lower our cholesterol levels, raising the HDL and preventing LDL (bad) cholesterol from building up on arterial walls. Although garlic's heart benefits may be new to some, for centuries herbalists have been using garlic to treat people with angina attacks and circulatory disorders.

Cayenne: Cayenne pepper is considered a "metabolism boosting herb" It is said that the main ingredient of cayenne pepper is capsaicin, which is a thermogenic chemical, that helps in speeding your metabolism and at the same time acts as an appetite suppressant. Not only can cayenne promote weight loss, but it is very high in vitamin A, C and the B complexes, also rich in calcium and potassium, helping to maintain a healthy circulatory and digestive system.

Replace Sugar and Honey with Agave Syrup
...a product of the new generation of healthy foods.

Introducing here 'AGAVE SYRUP" a product that is not found in recipes, as this is a product that we are just learning how to use; but is worth looking into the use of this product, because of its health benefits. Agave compared to other sweeteners has the lowest glycemic index, thus preventing sharp fluctuations in the blood sugar, which is the main cause in changes in mood, energy and hunger pangs.

Because many recipes do require a sweetener, what better way than to learn how to use Agave, a product that is not only delicious, but it has a smooth and thin texture mixing well with drinks, it goes well as a garnish for fruits and could be used in baking with the same results as sugar.

Where to find Agave? Supermarkets are starting to carry Agave Syrup, found usually next to the honey, or organic products, you can also find it in health food store and online. Check to make sure that it is "pure Agave" and does not contain any additives, if you can find "organic Agave" even better.

Agave contains, among other things, substances known as fructans, which are thought to reduce cholesterol, also containing, **Inulin,** a type of fructan, which is a carbohydrate found in many plants, including asparagus. *Some scientists believe inulin helps weight loss.*

Why replace sugar? The average American diet contains about 2 to 3 pounds of sugar per week, made up of refined sugar or table sugar, dextrose and corn syrups which are processed into many of the pre-packed foods such as breads, cereals, sauces and most microwavable foods. An excess of sugar triggers the release of insulin, which the body uses to keep blood-sugar at a constant and safe level. Insulin also promotes the storage of belly fat, so that when you eat sweets high in sugar, you're making way for rapid weight gain and elevated triglyceride levels, both of which have been linked to cardiovascular disease.

-10-

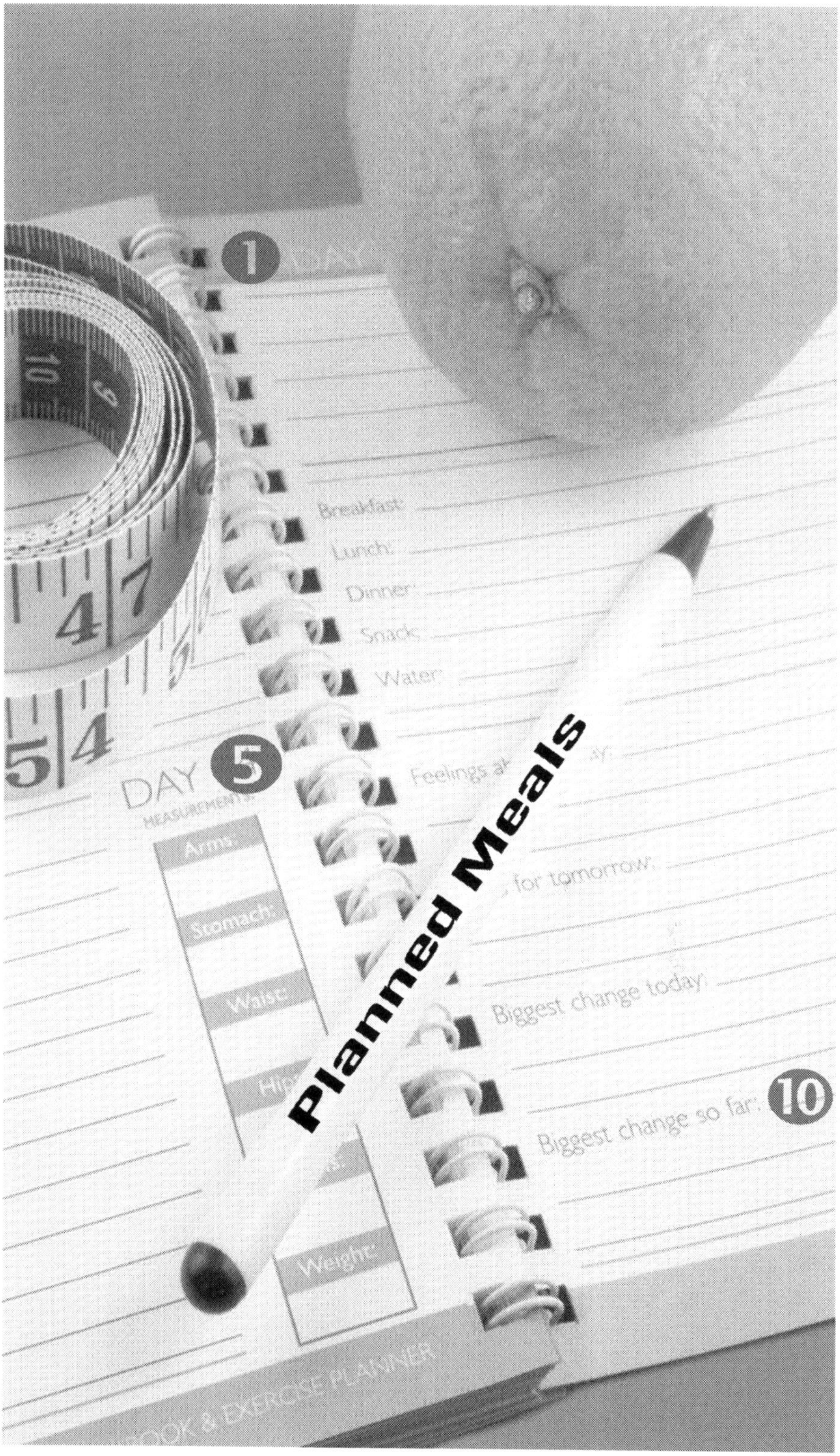

Planned Meals

Days 1 & 2

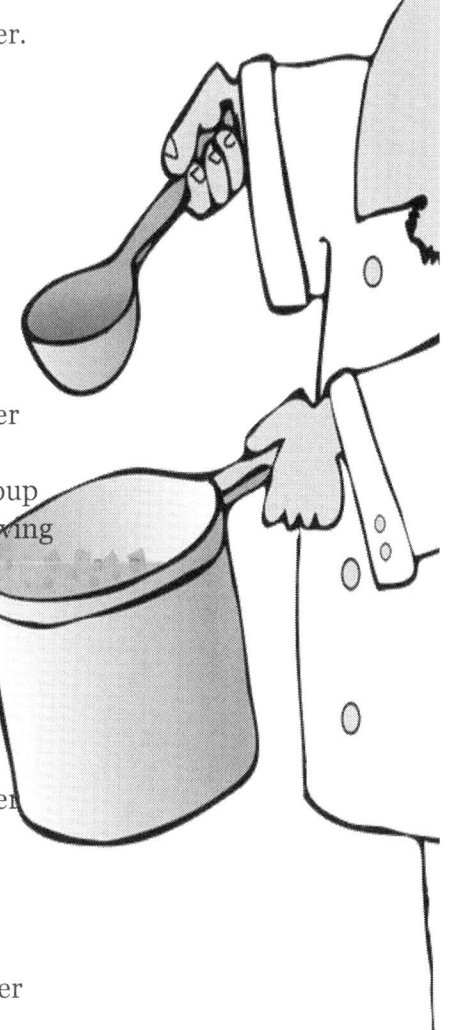

Breakfast:

- Any fruit, except bananas
- Coffee, tea
- Cranberry juice mixed with water.

Snack:

- Any of the yogurt drinks, recipes: pages 54-56
- green tea, or teas pages 52,53

Lunch:

- Soup Recipe #1 or #2
- Tea
- Cranberry juice mixed with water

Besides your lunch and dinner soup serving, you may have a soup serving any other time during the day

Snack:

- Any fruit, except bananas
- Tea
- Cranberry juice mixed with water

Dinner:

- Soup Recipe #1 or #2
- Tea
- Cranberry juice mixed with water

Besides your lunch and dinner soup serving, you may have a soup serving any other time during the day.

Planned Meals
Days 3 & 4

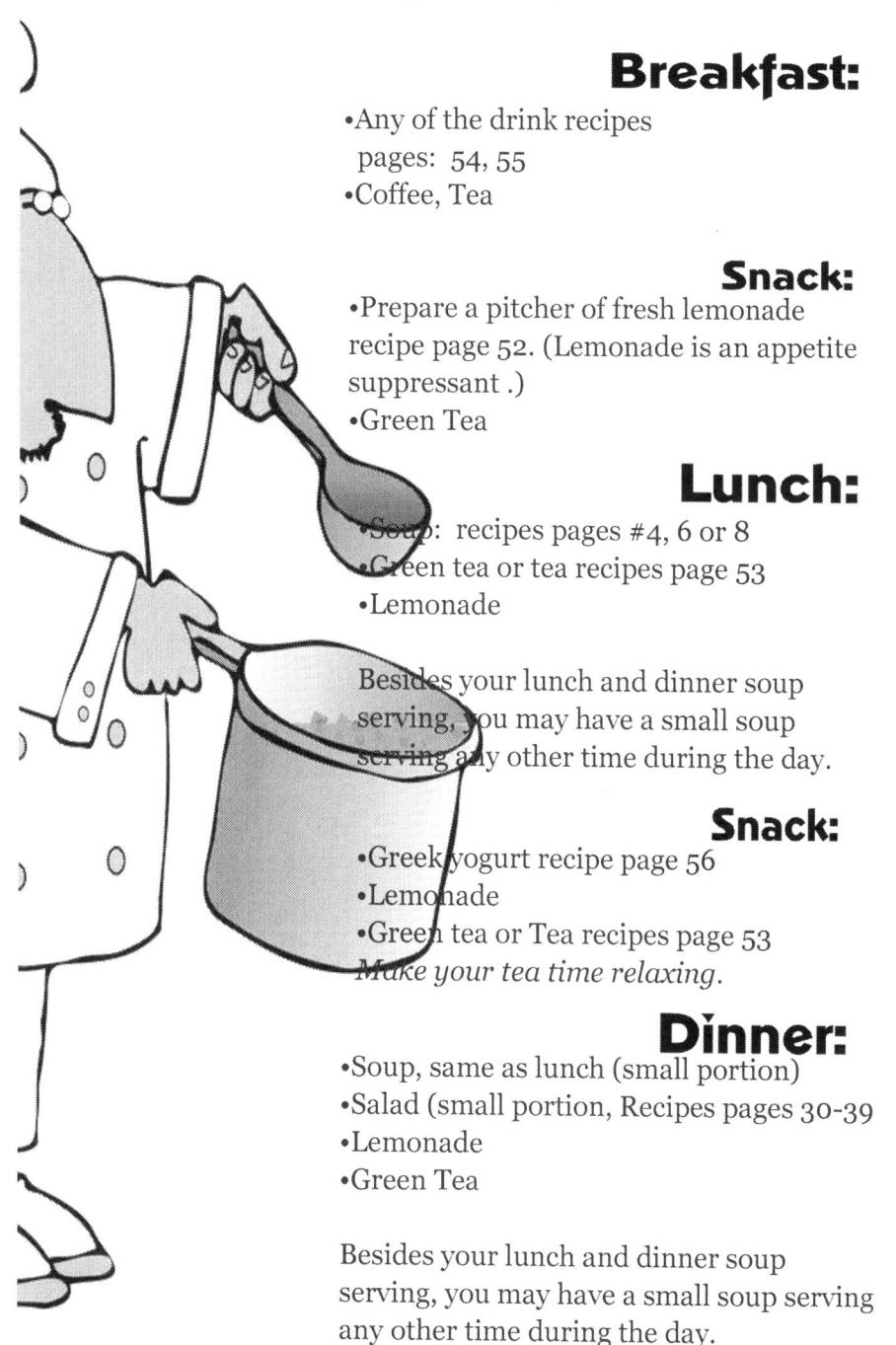

Breakfast:
- Any of the drink recipes pages: 54, 55
- Coffee, Tea

Snack:
- Prepare a pitcher of fresh lemonade recipe page 52. (Lemonade is an appetite suppressant .)
- Green Tea

Lunch:
- Soup: recipes pages #4, 6 or 8
- Green tea or tea recipes page 53
- Lemonade

Besides your lunch and dinner soup serving, you may have a small soup serving any other time during the day.

Snack:
- Greek yogurt recipe page 56
- Lemonade
- Green tea or Tea recipes page 53

Make your tea time relaxing.

Dinner:
- Soup, same as lunch (small portion)
- Salad (small portion, Recipes pages 30-39
- Lemonade
- Green Tea

Besides your lunch and dinner soup serving, you may have a small soup serving any other time during the day.

-13-

Planned Meals
Days 5 & 6

Breakfast:
Today is "banana day" it helps to control sugar cravings.
- Banana
- Coffee, Tea
- Cranberry juice mixed with water or lemonade

Snack:
- Banana
- Skim Milk or Almond Milk
- You can also prepare as a banana shake.

Lunch:
- Soup Recipe #3, 5, or 7
- Tea
- Cranberry juice mixed with water or lemonade.

Besides your lunch and dinner soup serving, you may have a small soup serving any other time during the day.

Snack:
- Greek yogurt, recipe page 56 top with a sliced banana.
- Green tea or tea recipes page 53.

Dinner:
- Soup, same as lunch
- Vegetable (small portion) Recipes pages 42-49
- Green tea or tea recipes page 53.
- Glass of cranberry juice mixed with water before bedtime.

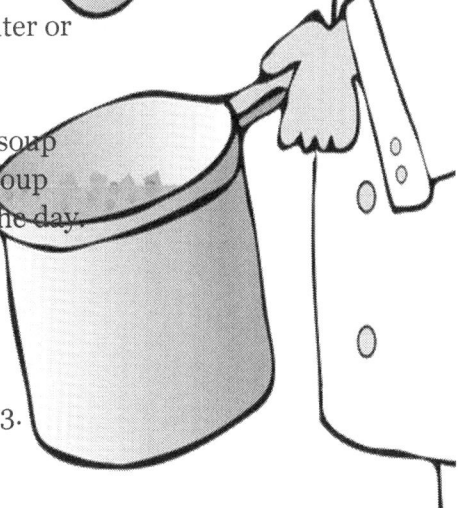

Besides your lunch and dinner soup serving, you may have a small soup serving any other time during the day.

Planned Meals
Days 7 & 8

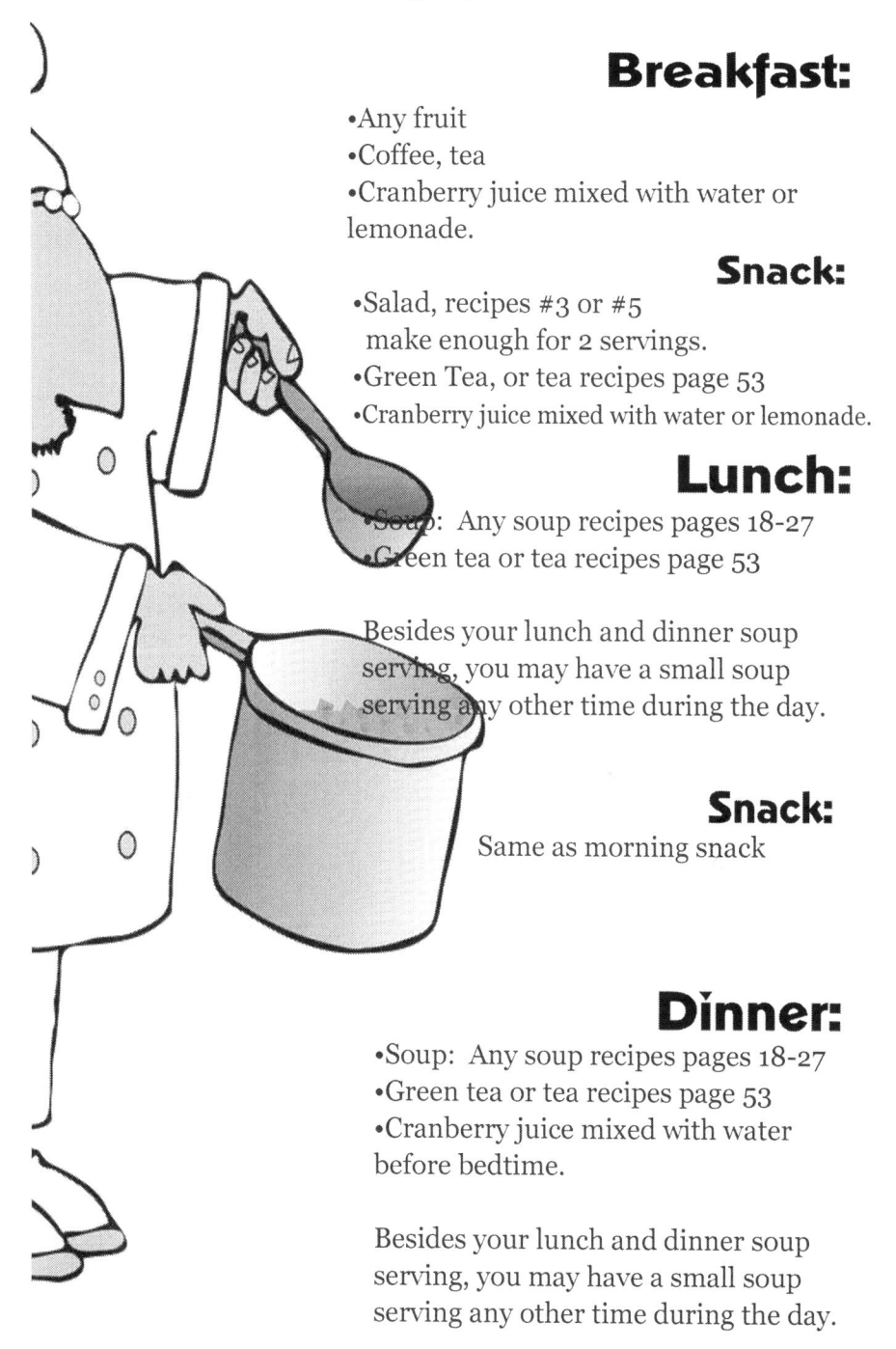

Breakfast:

- Any fruit
- Coffee, tea
- Cranberry juice mixed with water or lemonade.

Snack:

- Salad, recipes #3 or #5 make enough for 2 servings.
- Green Tea, or tea recipes page 53
- Cranberry juice mixed with water or lemonade.

Lunch:

- Soup: Any soup recipes pages 18-27
- Green tea or tea recipes page 53

Besides your lunch and dinner soup serving, you may have a small soup serving any other time during the day.

Snack:

Same as morning snack

Dinner:

- Soup: Any soup recipes pages 18-27
- Green tea or tea recipes page 53
- Cranberry juice mixed with water before bedtime.

Besides your lunch and dinner soup serving, you may have a small soup serving any other time during the day.

Planned Meals
Days 9 & 10

Breakfast:
- Any drink recipes pages 54, 55
- Coffee, tea

Snack:
- Any fruit
- Green tea or tea recipes page 53

Lunch:
- Soup: any soup recipe pages **18-27**
- Salad: small portion recipes pages **36-39**
- Green Tea
- Lemonade

Besides your lunch and dinner soup serving, you may have a small soup serving any other time during the day.

Snack:
- Any fruit, or
- Yogurt recipe page 56
- Green tea or tea recipes page 53

Dinner:
- Soup: any soup recipe pages 18-27
- Vegetable: small portion recipes pages 42-49
- Green Tea
- Lemonade

Besides your lunch and dinner soup serving, you may have a small soup serving any other time during the day.

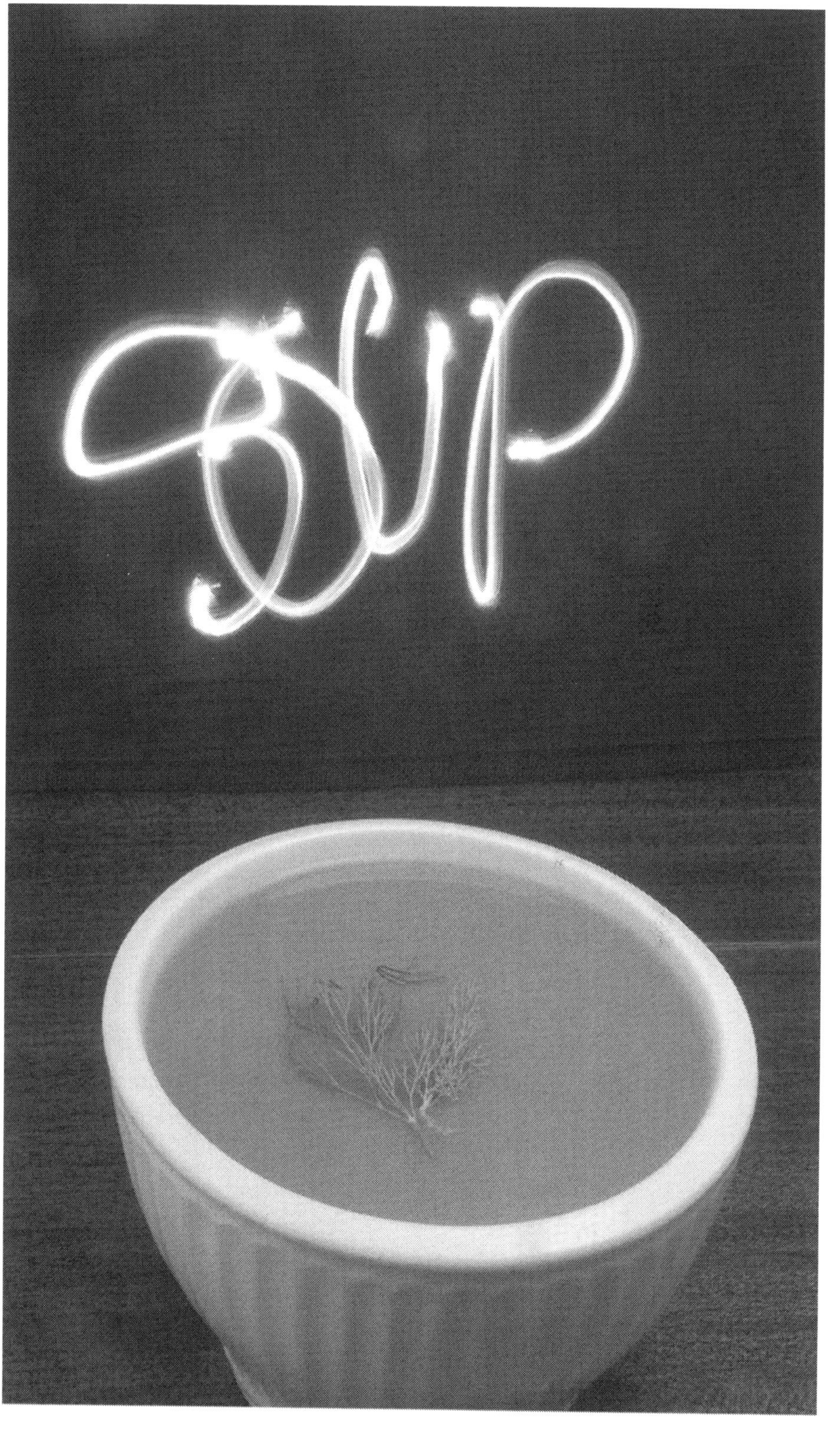

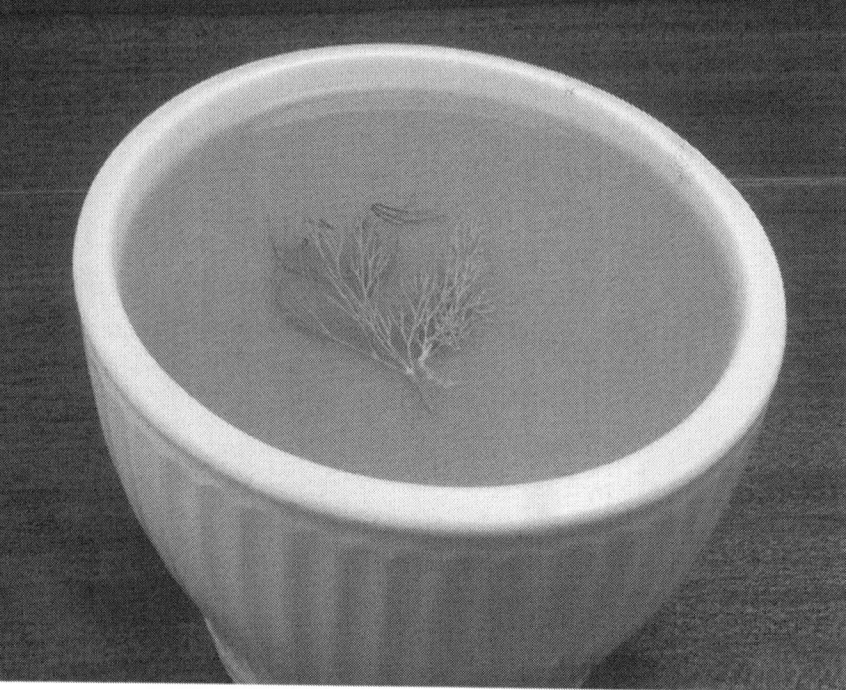

Mediterranean Style Cabbage and Vegetable Soup

Soup Recipe #1

This is a delicious and heart warming soup, that is easily made with any vegetables that you have on hand, feel free to improvise.

4 Servings, double the ingredients if you want to make it for 2 days.

Calories per serving: aprox. 45-50 calories.

Ingredients:
- 1 onion, chopped
- 2 garlic cloves, finely chopped
- 1 teaspoon virgin olive oil
- 2 small carrots, sliced
- 1 cup of green beans, chopped
- 2 medium tomatoes, chopped
- 3 cups of chopped cabbage
- 1 cup of chopped celery
- 8 cups of water
- Sea salt and pepper to taste

After serving, garnish with a tablespoon of parsley or cilantro, chopped finely.

Preparation:
In a large saucepan, heat oil over medium heat, sauté onion until starting to turn brown. Add tomatoes and continue to cook for a few more minutes, stirring frequently. Add all remaining ingredients, and bring to a boil, reduce heat and simmer partially covered for 25 to 35 minutes.

Many recipes for Cabbage soup in the internet calls for seasoning with bouillon cubes, V8 juice, or soup mixes. Do not consider any of these options for seasoning, as they are high in sodium and will cause you to retain water. *Nothing like natural seasoning!*

Cabbage and Beet Soup

Soup Recipe #2

This recipe is truly delicious, and is not in anyway to be considered a dieting soup, it just happens that is low in calories, and because of the cabbage and beets, it's a super "negative calories" soup. Enjoy!

4 Servings, double the ingredients if you want to make it for 2 days.

Calories per serving: aprox. 35-45 calories.

Ingredients:
- 1 onion, chopped
- 2 garlic cloves, finely chopped
- 1 teaspoon virgin olive oil
- 2 cups of sliced beets (you may used canned beets)
- 3 cups of chopped red cabbage
- 1 cup of chopped celery
- 8 cups of water
- 1/4 teaspoon oregano
- Sea salt and pepper to taste

ter serving, garnish with a tablespoon of parsley or cilantro, chopped finely.

Preparation:
In a large saucepan, heat oil over medium heat, sauté onion until starting to turn brown. Add garlic and continue to cook for a few more minutes, stirring frequently. Add all remaining ingredients, and bring to a boil, reduce heat and simmer partially covered for 25 to 35 minutes.

Tip: For delicious flavoring, make your soups over a sauté of onions, garlic, tomatoes, and your choice of spices, if you are using chicken or fish, add to your mix and sauté together for a few minutes, then add all other ingredients.

Cream of Tomato Skinny Soup

Soup Recipe #3

A delicious and elegant soup for any occasion.

4 Servings, double the ingredients if you want to make it for 2 days

Calories per serving: aprox. 65-75 calories

Ingredients:
- 6 ripe tomatoes, peeled, seeded, and chopped,
- 1 medium onion, chopped
- 1 tsp corn starch
- ¼ cup olive oil
- 2 garlic cloves
- 4 cups vegetable broth
- 1 tsp sun dried tomato paste
- 1/4 tsp oregano
- Sea salt and pepper to taste

Garnish:
- Plain yogurt or sour cream
- ¼ cup parsley, finely chopped

Preparation:

In a medium saucepan, start by adding the olive oil, onion and garlic, stirring until softened. Add a little of the vegetable broth and corn starch, stir until corn starch is dissolved, add the tomatoes, and the rest of the ingredients, and bring to a boil. Reduce heat to low, cover and simmer in low for about 15 minutes. Remove from heat, and let it cool a little.

In a food processor, puree the soup in batches until smooth. Return to saucepan and reheat for another 3 to 5 minutes.

Serve and garnish the soup with a tablespoon of yogurt or sour cream, sprinkle with the chopped parsley.

Hortosoupa – Vegetable Soup with Pasta

Soup Recipe #4

4 Servings, double the ingredients if you want to make it for 2 days.

Calories per serving: 65-75 calories (without the pasta)
Calories per serving: 100-110 calories (with the pasta)

This soup is easily made with any vegetables that you have on hand, feel free to improvise.

Ingredients:
- 1/4 cup of olive oil
- 1 onion, chopped
- 1 medium potato, cubed
- 2 small carrots, sliced
- 1 cup of green beans, chopped
- 2 zucchini, chopped
- 3 medium tomatoes, chopped
- 1 cup of chopped cabbage
- 1 cup of chopped celery
- 6 cups of water
- Sea salt and pepper to taste
- 1/2 cup of small orzo pasta (or other small soup pasta), **optional**

Preparation:

In a large saucepan, heat oil over medium heat, sauté onion until starting to turn brown. Add tomatoes and continue to cook for a few more minutes, stirring frequently. Add all remaining ingredients, except the pasta. Bring to a boil, reduce heat and simmer partially covered for 30 to 45 minutes. In the last 5 minutes before time is up, add pasta.

Cream of Broccoli Skinny Soup

Soup Recipe #5

4 Servings, double the ingredients if you want to make it for 2 days.

Calories per serving: 65-75 calories

Ingredients:
- 8 cups broccoli florets
- 1 onion, chopped
- 1 stalk celery, chopped
- 4 cups vegetable broth
- ¼ cup olive oil
- 1 tbsp fresh lemon juice
- ¼ tsp cumin
- 1 tbsp cornstarch
- Sea salt and black pepper to taste

Garnish:
- Plain yogurt or sour cream
- ¼ cup parsley, finely chopped

Preparation:
In a medium saucepan, start by adding the olive oil, and onion stirring until softened. Add a little of the vegetable broth and corn starch, stir until the cornstarch is dissolved, add the broccoli and the rest of the ingredients, and bring to a boil. Reduce head to low, cover and simmer in low for about 15 minutes. Remove from heat, and let it cool a little.

In a food processor, puree the soup in batches until smooth. Return to saucepan and reheat for another 3 to 5 minutes.

Serve and garnish the soup with a tablespoon of yogurt or sour cream, sprinkle with the chopped parsley.

The Skinny Fish Soup

Soup Recipe #6

This is a delicious and nutritious soup.

4 Servings, double the ingredients if you want to make it for 2 days.

Calories per serving: 100-120 calories (without the cheese)
Calories per serving: 120-150 calories   (with the cheese)

Ingredients:
- 1 large onion, finely chopped
- 1 green pepper, finely chopped
- 4 garlic cloves, minced
- 2 large ripe tomatoes, chopped
- ½ tsp oregano
- ½ tsp basil
- ¼ cup cilantro
- 1/2 cup cooking white wine
- 2 cups vegetable broth
- 1 pound white fish fillet (to taste)
- Sea salt and pepper to taste
- Grated parmesan cheese for garnish (optional)

Preparation:
In the olive oil sauté the onion, peppers, tomatoes, and garlic, to this mixture add the spices, wine and vegetable broth. Simmer for 10 minutes. Cut fish into chunks and add to soup, let it simmer for another 5 to 10 minutes until fish is cooked. Serve and sprinkle with the parmesan cheese. (optional)

Tip: Tilapia is an excellent choice of fish for this soup, as its tender and doesn't have a strong fishy taste.

Cream of Spinach Skinny Soup

Soup Recipe #7

4 Servings, double the ingredients if you want to make it for 2 days.

Calories per serving: 65-75 calories

Ingredients:
- 2 large packages of Spinach
- 1 onion, chopped
- 2 garlic cloves, minced
- 1 stalk celery, chopped
- 4 cups vegetable broth
- ¼ cup olive oil
- 1 tbsp fresh lemon juice
- ¼ tsp allspice (optional
- 1 tbsp cornstarch
- Sea salt and black pepper to taste

Garnish:
- Plain yogurt or sour cream
- ¼ cup parsley, for cilantro finely chopped

Preparation:
In a medium saucepan, start by adding the olive oil, and onion stirring until softened. Add a little of the vegetable broth and corn starch, stir until the cornstarch is dissolved, add the spinach and the rest of the ingredients, and bring to a boil. Reduce head to low, cover and simmer in low for about 15 minutes. Remove from heat, and let it cool a little.

In a food processor, puree the soup in batches until smooth. Return to saucepan and reheat for another 3 to 5 minutes.

Serve and garnish the soup with a tablespoon of yogurt or sour cream, sprinkle with the chopped parsley.

Cabbage, Carrot, & Pea Soup
Soup Recipe #8

4 Servings, double the ingredients if you want to make it for 2 days.

Calories per serving: 65-75 calories (without the pasta)
Calories per serving: 100-110 calories (with the pasta)

A simple, but delicious and filling skinny soup.

Ingredients:
- 1/4 cup of olive oil
- 1 onion, chopped
- 2 garlic cloves, minced
- 1 medium size package of frozen carrots and peas
- 3 cups chopped red cabbage
- 3 medium tomatoes, chopped
- 1 cup of chopped celery
- 6 cups of water
- Sea salt and pepper to taste
a pinch of cayenne (optional)
- 1/2 cup of small orzo pasta (or other small soup pasta), **optional**

Garnish with chopped cilantro before serving.

Preparation:
In a large saucepan, heat oil over medium heat, sauté onion and garlic until starting to turn brown. Add tomatoes and continue to cook for a few more minutes, stirring frequently. Add all remaining ingredients, except the pasta. Bring to a boil, reduce heat and simmer partially covered for 30 to 45 minutes. In the last 5 minutes before time is up, add pasta.

Chickpea Soup

Soup Recipe #9

Consider this soup during your Skinny Soup Dieting, as chickpeas are high in dietary fiber, manganese and B vitamins. The calorie content per serving is also low, or aprox. 60 calories per serving, when in soup.

4 Servings, double the ingredients if you want to make it for 2 days.

Calories per serving: 75-85 calories

Ingredients:
- 1 16 oz can chickpeas, drained and rinsed
- 5 cups vegetable stock
- 2 garlic cloves, crushed
- 1 hot pepper, finely chopped
- 1/4 cup cilantro, finely chopped
- 1/2 tsp oregano
- ½ tsp cumin
- Sea salt and pepper to taste

Garnish:
- 3 tbsp fresh lemon juice
- 3 Tbsp of olive oil
- ¼ cup cilantro, finely chopped
- 2 to 4 dry croutons per serving (optional) this adds an extra 10 calories.

Preparation:
In a medium saucepan add the chickpeas and vegetable stock and boil for 10 minutes, add the remaining ingredients except the garnish ingredients (olive oil, lemon juice, cilantro and croutons) continue to cook over medium heat another 10 minutes. Make a dressing with the garnish ingredients serve the soup and spoon in the center the garnishing dressing.

Vegetable White Bean Soup

Soup Recipe #10

Consider this soup during your Skinny Soup Dieting, as beans are high in dietary fiber, manganese and B vitamins. The calorie content per serving is also low, or aprox. 60 calories per serving, when in soup.

4 Servings, double the ingredients if you want to make it for 2 days.

Calories per servings: 80-90 Calories

Ingredients:
- 1 16 oz. can cannelloni or white beans, drained and rinsed
- 1 yellow onion chopped fine
- 2 large carrots cut into half inch pieces
- 2 stalks of celery
- 2 small bay leaves
- 2 leeks, finely chopped
- 2 tomatoes, finely chopped
- 3 garlic cloves, minced
- 6 cups of vegetable broth
- ¼ cup olive oil
- 2 tsp dried oregano
- 1/2 tsp paprika to taste
- Sea salt and pepper to taste

Garnish with chopped parsley or cilantro.

In the olive oil sauté the onions, tomatoes, garlic. Add the rest of the vegetables and spices, and let it simmer in the vegetable broth for 10 minutes, or until the vegetables are cooked.

Add the white beand to the vegetables adding more vegetable broth if it seems the soup is too thick. Cook for another 20 minutes.

Tip: To really get the flavor of the beans, use ¼ cup of beans and blend with ½ cup of water. Add this puree together with the beans before the last 20 minutes of cooking.

Personal Notes ♥

SALADS

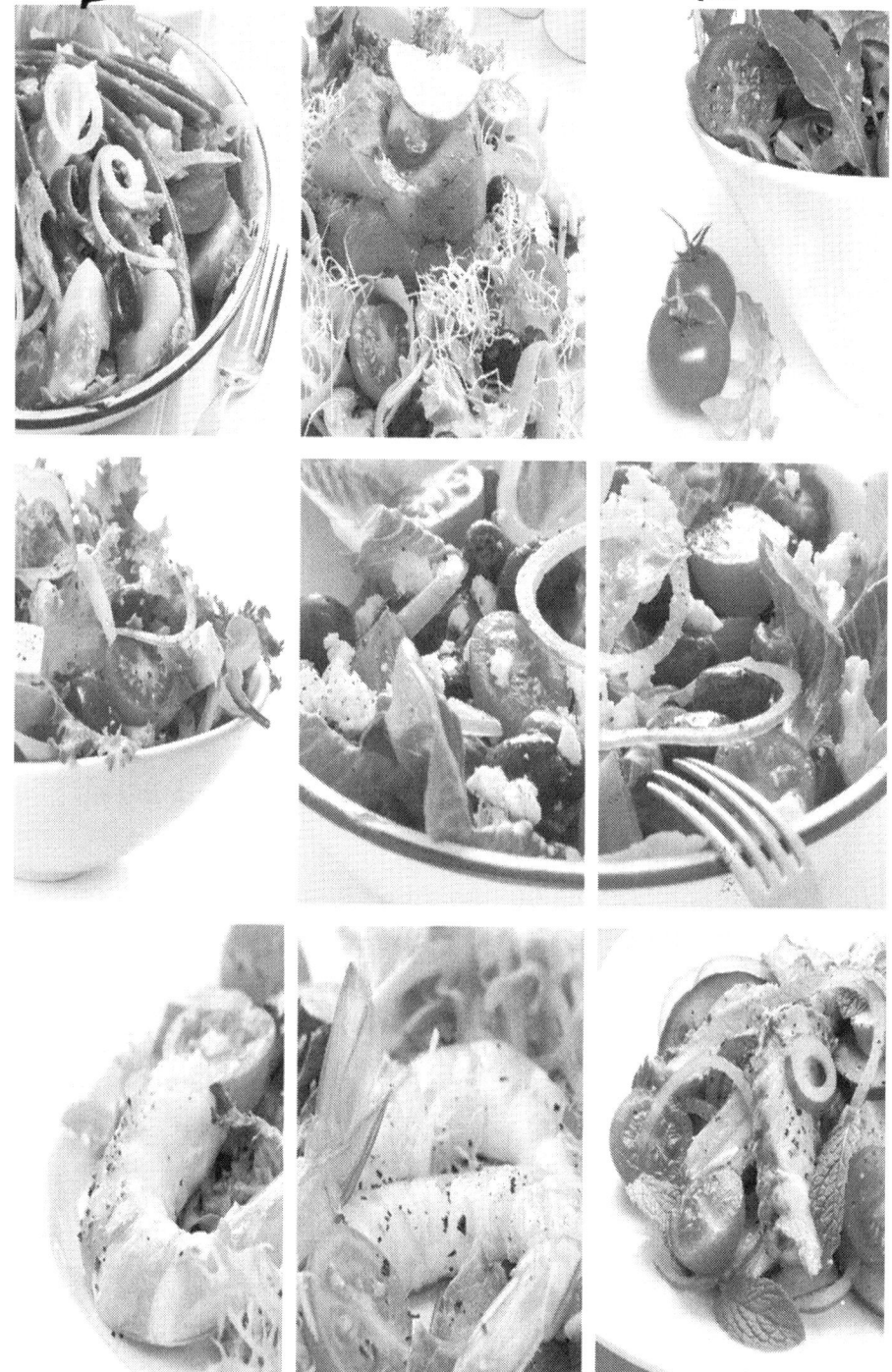

Cauliflower and Carrot Salad

Salad Recipe #1

4 Servings

Calories per serving: 75-80 calories

Ingredients:
- 1 Cauliflower head
- 2 carrots, cut in strips
- 1 small jar roasted red peppers, drained and cut in strips
- 8 black olives pitted and chopped
- 2 tbsp capers, drained and chopped
- ½ cup parsley, finely chopped

Dressing:
- 2 tbsp virgin olive oil
- 2 tbsp wine vinegar
- ¼ tsp (or less) cayenne (optional)
- Sea salt and black pepper to taste

Preparation:
In a saucepan filled with salted water bring to boil the cauliflower broken into small florets. Cook for 5-7 minutes, until barely tender. (do not over cook) Drain the cauliflower and combine in a bowl with all the ingredients, and pour over the dressing. Careful with the salt, as the capers and olives will add salt to the taste.

Beet and Yogurt Salad

Salad Recipe #2

4 Servings.

Calories per serving: 85-100 calories

Ingredients:
- 4 – 5 medium size beets, roasted (see how below)
- 1 1/2 Tbsp sherry or cider vinegar
- 1/2 Tsp Honey
- 2 Tbsp extra virgin olive oil
- Sea Salt
- Black pepper
- 1 to 2 garlic cloves
- 1/2 cup thick Greek style yogurt
- 2 Tbsp minced dill

Preparation:
Roast the beets, peel and cut into half moons.
In a bowl mix together the vinegar, honey, olive oil, and salt (low on the salt) and pepper to taste, toss in the warm beets and allow them to soak the flavors for 1 to 2 hours in the refrigerator.

Yogurt Dressing: Mash garlic to a paste, add a little salt, mix paste into the yogurt and add in half the dill.

Drain the beets and arrange on a platter and pour the yogurt over the top. Sprinkle the remaining dill.

How to roast beets:
Roasted beets have a sweeter flavor and easier to peel.
Preheat oven to 375*F Place washed beets in aluminum foil, sprinkle with olive oil, and seal the foil. (all the beets you are roasting in one foil package) Bake until tender from 30-45 minutes.
Let them cool enough to handle and peel.

Pomegranate and Almond Salad

Salad Recipe #3

4 Servings

Calories per serving: 65-85 calories

This is a delicious and simple salad, bursting with the exotic flavor of the pomegranate and sweet almonds.

Ingredients:
- 1 head of romaine lettuce
- 1/2 lb watercress (2 bunches), coarse stems discarded and sprigs cut into 1-inch pieces (6 cups)
- 1 carrot - grated
- Seeds from 1 large pomegranate (1 -1/4 cups), white membranes discarded
- 3/4 cup sliced almonds , toasted
- 1 Tsp Honey

Dressing:
- 2 tablespoons fresh lemon juice
- 3 Tbsp virgin olive oil
- Sea salt to taste
- Black pepper to taste

Preparation:
Toast almonds in a saucepan over medium heat. Toast by stirring constantly, once you see they begin to toast add the honey. Remove from heat and let them cool.

Combine lettuce, watercress, grated carrot, and the pomegranate seeds in a large serving bowl. Add dressing and mix. Serve and sprinkle with the toasted almonds.

Mediterranean Salad

Salad Recipe #4

4 Servings

Calories per serving: 85-100 calories

Ingredients:
- 1 head lettuce or assortment of salad greens of your choice (arugula, radicchio etc...)
- 3 cucumbers, seeded and sliced
- 1 cup crumbled feta cheese
- 1 cup black olives, pitted and sliced
- 3 cups diced tomatoes
- 1/3 cup diced sun-dried tomatoes, drained
- 1/2 red onion, sliced

Dressing:
- 3 Tbsp virgin olive oil
- ¼ cup fresh lemon juice
- 2 garlic cloves minced
- ½ cup parsley
- Sea Salt
- Cumin
- Black Pepper

Preparation:
In a salad bowl, mix together all the ingredients, except the ingredients for the dressing. Chill until ready to serve, pour the dressing before serving.

Zesty Vegetable & Fruit Salad

Salad Recipe #5

4 Servings

Calories per serving: 85-100 calories

Ingredients:
- 1 head of lettuce or assortment of salad greens (arugula, radicchio, lettuce)
- 3 tomatoes, sliced in quarters
- 1 cup mushrooms, thinly sliced
- 6 radishes, thinly sliced
- 1 large red pepper, sliced
- ½ cup almonds, sliced
- ½ cup green apple, sliced
- ½ cup oranges, chopped in small pieces

Dressing:
- ¼ cup virgin olive oil
- 3 tbsp orange juice
- 1 tbsp red vinegar
- ¼ tsp honey
- ¼ tsp paprika
- Sea salt to taste

In a large salad bowl, toss together all the ingredients. Pour over the dressing and serve.

White Beans and Tuna Salad

Salad Recipe #6

4 Servings

Calories per serving: 120-150 calories

A nutritious and delicious dish, served as a light main course.

Ingredients:
- 1 can of white beans, drained and rinsed
- 1 8oz can white tuna in olive oil
- 1 tbls caper, drained and dried
- 3 tbsp olive oil
- 1 tbsp red wine vinegar
- ¼ tbsp oregano
- ¼ cup parley, finely chopped
- 1 red onion, finely sliced
- Sea salt and pepper to taste

Preparation:
In a saucepan boil the white beans for 2 minutes, drain and transfer to a serving bowl ready with all the other ingredients, mix well.

Serve while the beans are still warm, or at room temperature.

Spinach Salad

Salad Recipe #7

4 Servings

Calories per serving: 75-90 calories

Ingredients:
- 1 lb baby spinach (4 to 5 cups spinach leaves)
- 6 cherry tomatoes cut in half
- 1 small red onion, thinly sliced
- 1 small jar roasted red peppers, cut in strips
- ¼ cup crumbled feta cheese
- ¼ cup walnuts, roasted

Dressing
- 3 Tbsp virgin olive oil
- ¼ cup fresh lemon juice
- ¼ tsp cumin
- Sea salt and pepper to taste

In a large salad bowl mix all the ingredients and top with dressing.

To roast walnuts: In a baking sheet at 350*F roast until slightly brown.

Zucchini Salad

Salad Recipe #8

4 Servings

Calories per serving: 85-100 calories

Ingredients:
- 1 Lb zucchini, cut in long strips
- 2 red peppers, cut in long strips
- 1/2 cup green olives, sliced
- 1/2 cup red onions
- 5 garlic cloves, minced
- 1 Tbsp olive oil
- 1 tsp thyme

Dressing:
- 2 tbsp capers, rinsed and drained
- 1/4 cup virgin olive oil
- 2 tbsp red wine or red wine vinegar
- 1/4 tsp allspice

Preparation:
In a large frying pan heat the olive oil, and at medium heat add the zucchini, red peppers, salt, black pepper, and sauté for 5 minutes. Remove from heat and add the rest of the ingredients, let it chill for 2 to 3 hours and before serving pour dressing.

Sauces & Dressings

Garlic Sauce

Optional changes for your salads

Ingredients:
- 6 garlic cloves, finely crushed
- ¼ tsp sea salt
- 2 tbsp virgin olive oil
- 3 tbsp fresh lemon juice

Preparation:
Combine all the ingredients together, and mix well. This dressing is for garlic lovers. Serve on the side for those that want a little more garlic taste to their salads or vegetable dishes.

Vinaigrette

Ingredients:
- ½ tsp mustard
- 2 tbsp red wine vinegar
- ½ cup virgin olive oil
- ½ tsp sea salt
- ¼ tsp black pepper

Preparation:
Mix all the ingredients until thoroughly dissolved. The use of a wire whisk is recommended.

Delicious with a simple fresh tomato and cheese salad, or plain green salads.

Tahini Sauce

Ingredients:
- 1 cup of tahini
- 1 tbsp olive oil
- 2 tbsp water (if required)
- ¼ cup fresh lemon juice
- 2 garlic cloves, minces
- ¼ tsp sea salt

Preparation:
In a food processor blend all the ingredients. If too thick add a little water, until desired consistency.

Great over salads containing chicken or tuna.

Yogurt and Mint Sauce

Ingredients:
- 2 cups plain Greek yogurt
- 2 garlic cloves, minced
- 2 tbsp fresh lemon juice
- 1 tbsp virgin olive oil
- ¼ cup fresh mint, finely chopped
- ¼ cup fresh parsley, finely chopped
- Sea salt to taste. (low on the salt)

Puree all the ingredients in a blender. Refrigerate if not using right away.

Try it with a spinach or beet salad.

Personal Notes

VEGETABLES

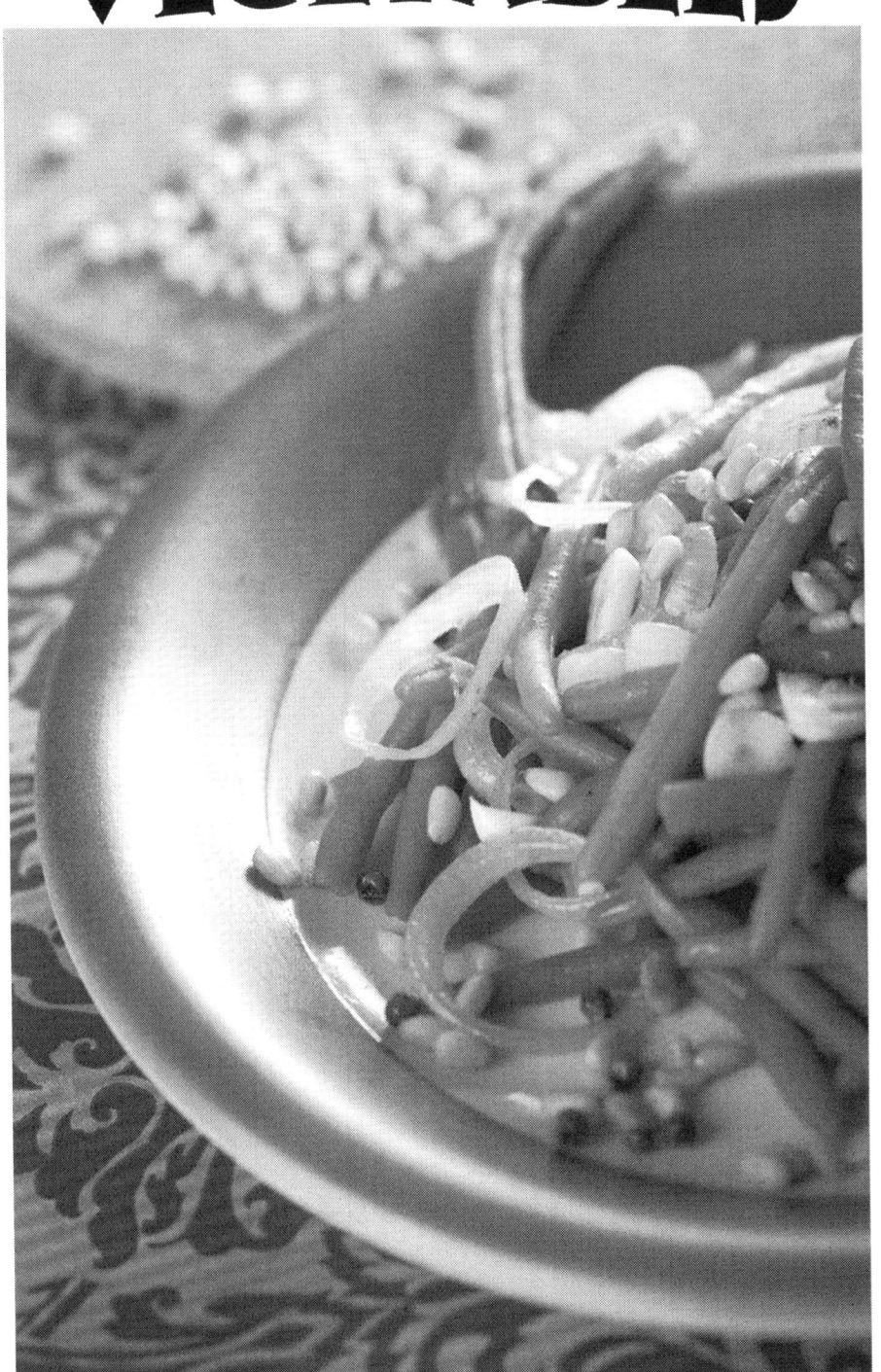

Cauliflower with Tahini

Vegetable Recipe #1

4 Servings

Calories per serving: 100-120 calories

Ingredients:
- 2 heads of cauliflower
- 2 Tsp Olive oil
- ¼ cup tahini
- 2 garlic cloves
- ½ cup fresh lemon juice
- ¼ cup vegetable stock
- Sea Salt to taste

Preparation
In a large skillet over medium heat, sauté the cauliflower in the olive oil for 10-12 minutes.

Mix the other ingredients in a separate bowl and add to the sautéed cauliflower. Cook the mixture for another 5-7 minutes.

About Tahini:
Tahini is a tick paste made of sesame seeds. It is an excellent source of manganese, copper, calcium, magnesium, iron, phosphorus, vitamin B1, zinc and dietary fiber. Sesame have shown to have cholesterol lowering effects and to prevent high blood pressure. Sesame seeds are also a good source of the amino acid Methionine, which is an important contributor to liver detoxification.

Baked Grilled Tomatoes

Vegetable Recipe #2

2-4 Servings

Calories per serving: 80-110

Ingredients:
- 4 small tomatoes
- 4 Tbsp Greek yogurt
- 1 glove of garlic
- 1 teaspoon dried basil, crushed
- 1 tablespoon fine dry bread crumbs
- 1 tablespoon finely shredded or grated Parmesan cheese
- Sea Salt to taste
- Pepper to taste

Preparation:
Preheat oven to 350*F
Cut tomatoes in half crosswise and remove insides carefully. Place cut to tomatoes on aluminum foil covered baking pan.

Mix Yogurt with minced garlic, salt (low on the salt) and pepper.
Fill tomatoes first with yogurt mixture, followed by a sprinkle of basil, bread crumbs and parmesan cheese.

Bake uncovered for 15 to 20 minutes.

Green Beans

Vegetable Recipe #3

4 Servings

Calories per serving: 100-110 calories

Ingredients:
- 2 lbs fresh green beans
- 1 onion, chopped
- 1/4 cup tomato paste
- 1 minced garlic clove
- 1 teaspoon fresh parsley, chopped
- 2 Tbsp olive oil
- 1 teaspoon salt
- 1/4 tsp black pepper
- ¼ tsp of cumin
- 2 cups water or vegetable broth

Preparation:
Clean and cut green beans, to bite sizes.
Saute the onions, garlic in 2 Tbsp of olive oil.
Mix the tomato paste, salt, pepper and cumin with 1 cup of water or stock.
Put all ingredients into a medium saucepan, cover and cook on low to medium heat until tender, stirring frequently for about 15 to 20 minutes.

Spinach, Chickpeas and Yogurt

Vegetable Recipe #4

4 Servings

Calories per serving: 100-120 calories

Ingredients
- 4 bunches or 4 packages of Spinach
- 1-16oz. can of chickpeas, drained and rinsed
- 2 large yellow onions
- 3 garlic cloves
- ½ cup parsley
- 1 tsp cumin
- ½ cup Greek Yogurt
- Sea Salt to taste
- Pepper to taste

Preparation:
In a large pot over medium heat sauté the onions with the 2 garlic cloves for 5 minutes. Add the washed and drained spinach, and sprinkle with the cumin, salt and pepper, (low on the salt) adding the parsley and mix well. Simmer for 10 minutes, add the chickpeas, stir, and simmer for another 5 minutes.

Yogurt dressing:
Minced 1 garlic clove, and mix with the yogurt, adding salt to taste.

Serve yogurt dressing separate to be use as a topping for the Spinach and Chickpea Dish.

Red Peppers with Mushrooms

Vegetable Recipe #5

4 Servings

Calories per serving: 80-100 calories

Ingredients:
- 2 red peppers, chopped
- 3 cups mushrooms, sliced
- 6 cherry tomatoes, cut in half
- 2 tbsp olive oil
- 3 garlic cloves, minced
- ¼ tsp allspice
- Sea salt and black pepper to taste

Preparation:
In a large skillet heat olive oil over medium heat, sauté peppers, garlic for about 7 minutes, add the tomatoes, mushrooms and spices, simmer covered for another 5 to 10 minutes.

Sautéed Mushrooms

Vegetable Recipe #6

3-4 Servings

Calories per serving: 80-100 calories

Ingredients:
- 12 whole mushrooms, cut in half.
- 2 garlic cloves, minced
- 2 tbsp olive oil
- ½ cup parsley, finely chopped
- Sea salt and black pepper to taste

Preparation:
In a frying pan heat the olive oil over medium heat, add the mushrooms, stirring constantly until they are tender, about 7 to 10 minutes. Add the minced garlic, salt, pepper and chopped parsley and continue stirring for another minute or two, being careful that the garlic doesn't burn.

Serve hot, as an entrée or side dish.

Asparagus with Almonds

Vegetable Recipe #7

4 Servings

Calories per serving: 100-120 calories

Ingredients:
- 2 lb or about 20 pcs Asparagus, trimmed
- ¼ cup olive oil
- 4 garlic cloves,
- 4 cup blanched almonds
- ½ cup bread crumbs
- 1 tbps sherry vinegar
- 3/4 cup vegetable broth, boiling hot
- Sea salt and black pepper to taste

Preparation:
Preheat oven to 400* F

Step one: In a saucepan heat 2 tbsp of the olive oil, add the garlic, almonds and bread crumbs and sauté stirring frequently, until they turn brown. (careful not to burn)

Step two: Transfer sautéed ingredients to a blender, add vinegar, salt, pepper and blend until it forms a thick mixture.

Step three: In the oil left in the saucepan, (you may add a little more olive oil) sauté the asparagus until they start to become tender, about 5 minutes.

Get ready for the oven: Place the asparagus in a glass oven dish, pour the hot vegetable broth and top with the almond-bread mixture. Bake for 15 to 20 minutes until the asparagus are cooked and most of the liquid has dried.

From the oven to the table! Serve immediately.

Italian Sweet and Sour Carrots

Vegetable Recipe #8

4 Servings

Calories per serving: 110-120 calories

Ingredients:
- 1 lb package baby carrots, peeled ready to eat type
- ½ lb about 12 baby onions, peeled
- ¼ cup olive oil
- 3 tbsp red wine vinegar
- 1 tbsp honey
- sea salt and black pepper
- 2 tbsp parsley

Preparation:
In a medium saucepan fill with lightly salted boiling water, cook for about 3 to 5 minutes, just to tenderize the carrots slightly. In a separate saucepan add the olive oil and cook the onions, for about 5 minutes, stirring frequently, add the carrots, black pepper and ¼ cup of the water where you boiled the carrots. Cook in low-medium for about 5 more minutes, and then add the vinegar, and honey, stir constantly until the liquid turns into a small amount of syrup. Serve hot, and garnish with the parsley.

Personal Notes ❤

DRINKS & SNACKS

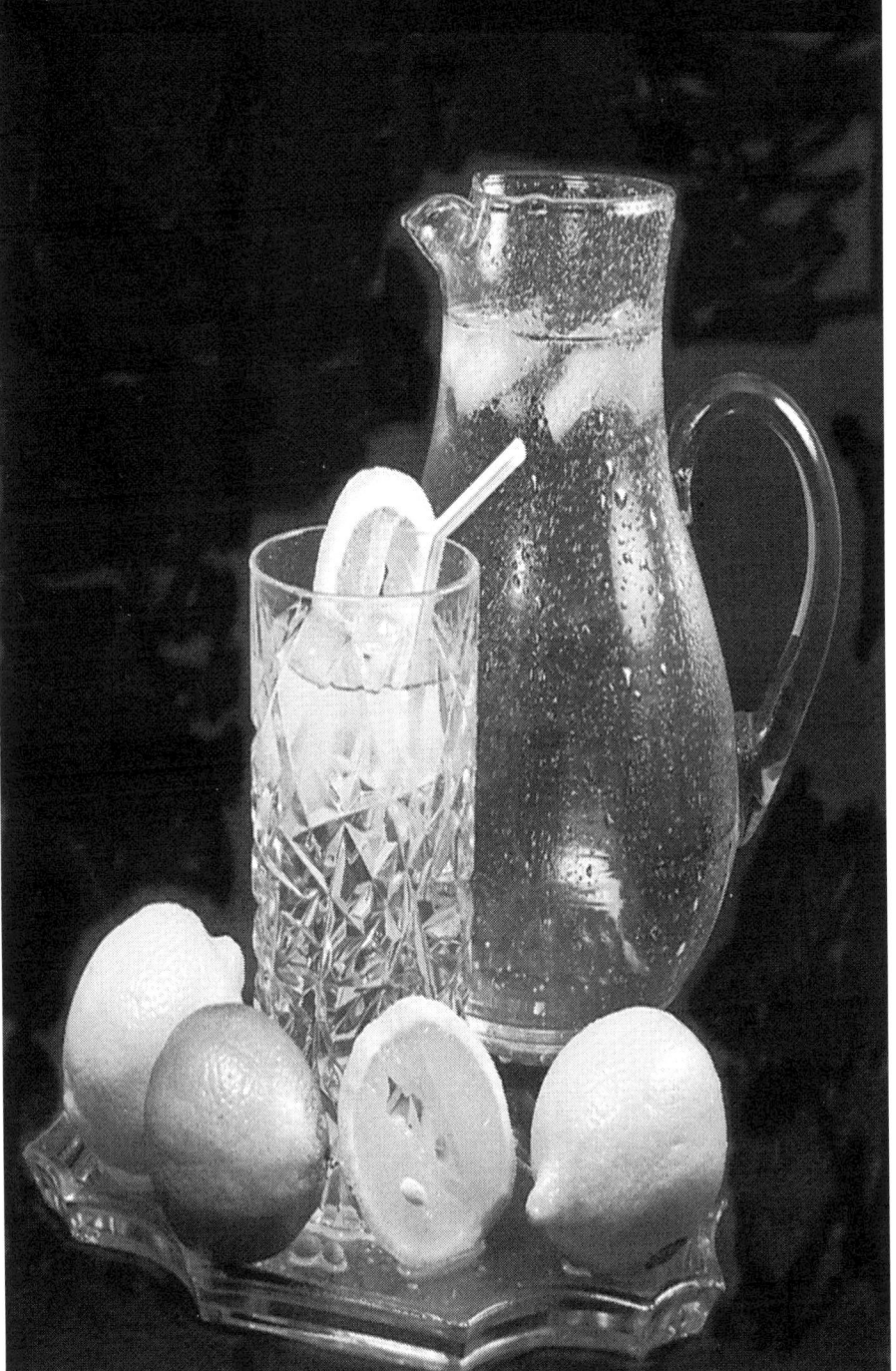

Lemonade

Not just lemonade! This is a refreshing and tasty way of making lemonade.

Ingredients:
- 8 fresh lemons
- 4 tbsp Agave Syrup
- 2 teaspoon orange blossom water
- 4 cups fresh finely chopped mint
- 8 cups of cold water

Blend all the ingredients together. Serve in tall glasses filled with crushed ice. Keep refrigerated until ready to serve.

Note: Please don't replace the Agave with substitute sugars, as these are full of chemicals. Agave is a natural sweetener, low in calories, low in glucose levels and well tolerated if you have concerns with sugar.

Benefits of Lemons

- They are rich in vitamins C, B and P.
- They help to fight bacteria and infections.
- They contain high levels of potassium, which regulates heart function and reduces blood pressure.
- They are considered alkaline helping problems with stomach acidity and digestion.

Note: *Lemons are the main ingredient in "The Lemonade Diet" a detox diet which recommends a mixture of lemons in water sweetened with maple syrup. A pinch of cayenne is usually added for its cleansing effects, with the added benefit of helping you to lose weight.*

Cinnamon Anise Tea

This is a wonderful tea for after dinner, or cold nights. The sweet licorice taste from the anise seeds gives this tea and exotic flavor.

Ingredients:
- 3 cups water
- 2 teaspoons anise seeds
- 2 sticks of cinnamon
- 1 1/2 tablespoon lemon juice
- 2 tbsp of Honey or 1 tbsp of Agave
- 2 black tea bags

Preparation:
Combine all the ingredients except the tea bags in a small pan (one that you use only for boiling water) and bring to boil. After it boils, add the tea bags. Allow to simmer for 2-3 minutes, strain and serve hot in glasses. You may garnish with a twist of lemon peel.

Lemon Tea
The secret is in the preparation of the tea!

Something as simple as tea can turn into a comforting and enjoyable moment.

Ingredients:
- 4 cups boiling water
- 4 tea bags
- 2 teaspoons of grated lemon peel
- 1 teaspoon lemon juice
- Honey as a sweetener (optional)

Preparation:
Boil water first and then add lemon peel, lemon juice and tea bags. Allow to steep for 10 minutes.

Yogurt and Fruit Drink

A refreshing drink for breakfast or a midday snack.

Calories per serving: 120-140

Ingredients:
- 10-15 Raspberries
- Small banana, peeled and sliced
- 3 tbsp of Agave
- 1 tsp lemon juice
- 3 tbsp plain low fat yogurt
- 1 cup low fat milk

Preparation:
Puree all ingredients in your blender or food processor. Serve in tall glasses with ice cubes.
A healthy way to start your day!

Yogurt and Orange Drink

Calories per serving: 100-110

Ingredients:
- 2 cups plain low fat yogurt
- 2 cups of orange juice
- 1 orange
- 1 tsp Agave
- 8 ice cubes

Blend together the yogurt, honey and orange juice, together with a small piece about 1 inch of orange peel. Blend until well mixed. Add the ice cubed and blend for another 30 seconds.

Pour into tall glasses, and garnish with an orange twist.

Strawberry Almond Shake

Calories per serving: 100-110 calories

Ingredients:
- 2 cups of almond low fat milk
- 2 cups of frozen strawberries
- 2 tbsp honey or agave
- ¼ tsp vanilla extract (optional)

Preparation:
Put all the ingredients in your blender, and mix until smooth. Preferably that you use frozen strawberries to give your shake a frozen finish, but if you use fresh strawberries, suggest that you add ½ cup crush ice to your shake. Serve in a tall glass.

Apple Milk Shake

Calories per serving: 80-100 calories

This is a Mediterranean drink, very refreshing and at the same time healthy. Something different to try.

Ingredients:
- 2 sweet apples, peeled and finely chopped
- 2 cups of low fat cold milk
- 1 tbsp honey or agave, (see page 17 for information about Agave)
- 1 tbsp rose water
- Crushed ice

Preparation:
Put all the ingredients in your blender, and mix until smooth. Serve in a tall glass over crushed ice.

Yogurt with Agave

Calories per serving: 100-110 calories

A delicious serving for breakfast, a snack during the day or served as a desert after a light meal.

Ingredients:
- 1/2 cup of Greek yogurt per serving
- 1-2 teaspoons of Agave per serving

Crushed pistachios and/or almonds (optional)

Preparation:
In individual serving bowls, drizzle Agave over the yogurt and sprinkle with crushed pistachios or almonds if desired.

Optional toppings:

- 1/2 sliced banana
- 2 large strawberries, sliced.

or

- 1/4 cup blueberries or raspberries

Drizzle fruit with Agave. Just delicious!

Tips to satisfy your need for something sweet

Not a very original recipe, but keeping sugar free gelatin prepared and ready for moments of weakness really helps. You can always add a few pieces of fruit, and top with a few drops of Agave, the satisfaction is in the sweetness and knowing that its only 20 calories or less per serving.

Red grapes are not only nutritious, but frozen grapes make a very satisfying snack. Grapes are little high in calories, so don't over do it; half of cup is about 50 calories.

Plain Greek style yogurt, is always an "I'm starving" saver, just add some fruit, nuts and drizzle with Agave. Delicious and nutritious!

Not really hungry, just a habit of thinking of food? Go for a nice cup of tea, green tea is not only healthy, but it will help you to lose the weight. Not in a mood for green tea, then make yourself a nice cup of tea from the recipes found on page 53.

Keep a bottle of prepared lemonade in the refrigerator. Lemonade is not only healthy, but it is an appetite suppressant. *This is the secret of The Lemonade Diet.*

OTHER DIETS DEFINED

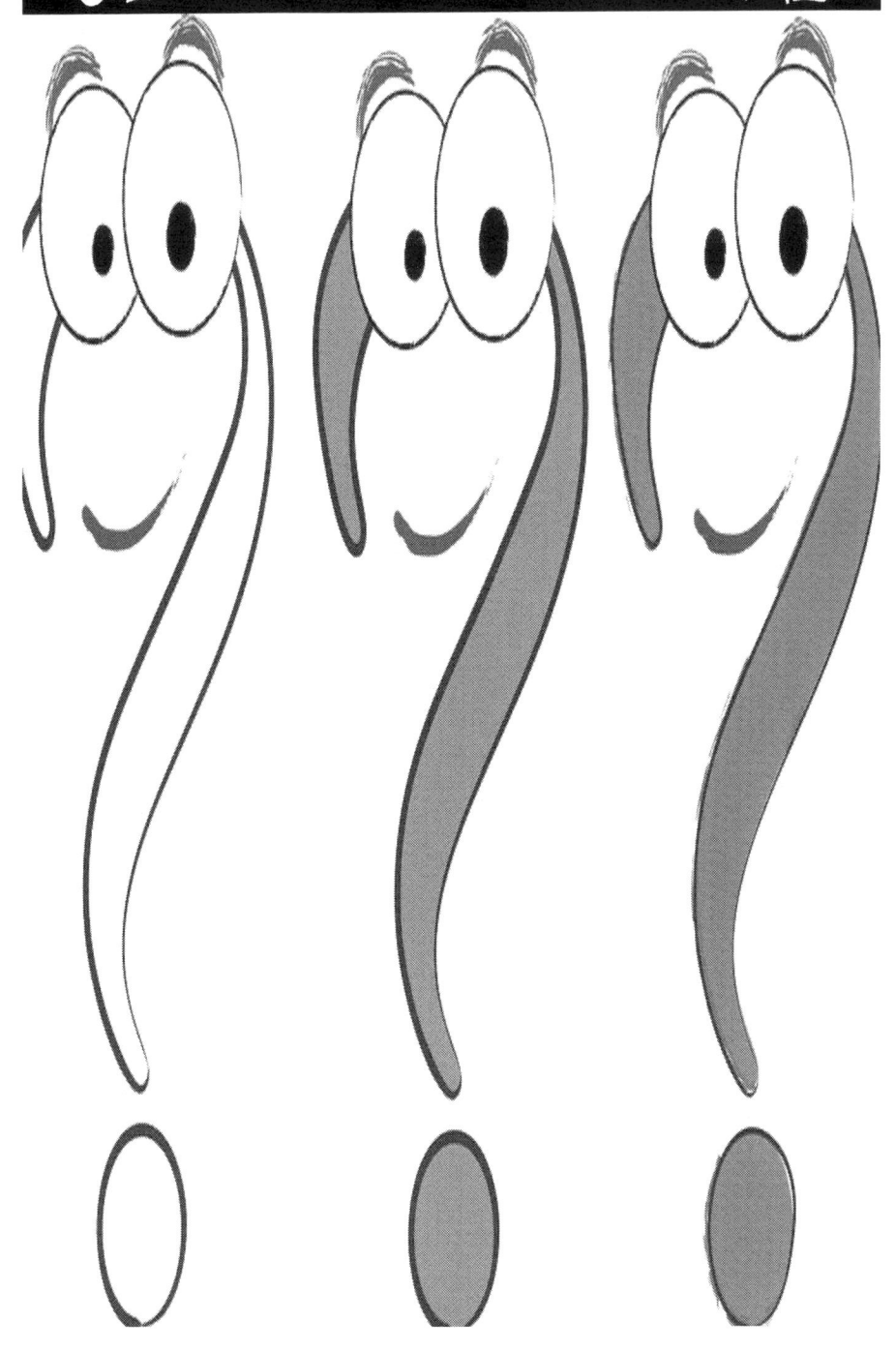

Which Diet is Yours?

We all know how difficult it's to decide which diet to follow, and to have the will power and commitment to follow a diet. Here you find a brief description of different diets. Some are easy, like the Mediterranean Diet, and you also find detox-diets, which are really considered fasting diets, like The Lemonade Diet.

The Mediterranean Diet defined: Decades ago, it was the natural way of life of people from countries bordering the Mediterranean Sea, countries including; Spain, France, Italy, Greece, Portugal and North Africa. The similarity in eating habits of these countries is what is referred as the Mediterranean Diet, which consist of: Lots of fruits and veggies, whole grain breads, beans, nuts, seeds. fish and poultry, very little meat, limited consumption of eggs, and red wine.

The Master Cleanse Diet, or as popularly known; *The Lemonade Diet* was created by the late Naturopath Stanley Burroughs. Strictly speaking, it's not a fast but a liquid-diet detox/cleanse. The mental craving for food passes quickly, and while toxins may be 'stired up' temporarily, they also will pass out of the body quickly. As a reducing diet it is superior in every way, reducing at a rate of about two (2) pounds a day for most persons, without harmful side effects. How much weight is lost will be greatly determined by how much syrup is used, but the detoxification will happen regardless.

Juicing: Juice therapy known as juicing involves extracting the juice from raw fruit and vegetables. From the 1970s on, Jay Kordich popularized the concept of drinking fresh juice to boost energy, lose weight, and for the healing results by following this form of diet. Clinical studies has shown that a diet rich in fruit and vegetables reduces the risk of such diseases such as heart disease, cancer, and diabetes.

South Beach Diet: The South Beach Diet is a diet plan designed by cardiologist Arthur Agatston and dietician Marie Almon as an alternative to low-fat diet approach The South Beach Diet is relatively simple in principle. It replaces "bad carbs" and "bad fats" with "good carbs" and "good fats." According to Agatston, hunger cycles are triggered not by carbohydrates in general, but by carbohydrate-rich foods that the body digests quickly, creating a spike in blood sugar. The South Beach Diet was designed by a cardiologist, it should be no surprise that it eliminates trans-fats and discourages saturated fats. Although foods rich in these "bad fats" do not contribute to the hunger cycle, they do contribute to LDL cholesterol and heart disease.

Atkins Diet: This diet involves the restriction of carbohydrates in order to switch the body's metabolism from burning glucose to burning stored body fat. This process called lipolysis begins when the body enters the state of ketosis as a consequence of running out of excess carbohydrates to burn.

Agave Master Cleanser: this is a modified detox diet, introduced by the creators of The Lemonade Diet . com where the ingredients of the Master Cleansers have been modified to the specific needs of pre diabetics or type 2 Diabetics.

Macrobiotic Diet: Is a dietary regimen which involves eating grains as a staple food supplemented with other local foodstuffs such as vegetables and beans. Macrobiotics also addresses the manner of eating by recommending against overeating and requiring that food be chewed thoroughly before swallowing.

Grapefruit Diet: The diet significantly limits the amount of fruits and vegetables one eats while encouraging meat intake; the combination of these high-fat, high-cholesterol foods with grapefruit is claimed to burn fat. A 2004 study funded by The Florida Citrus Department found that participants lost an average of 3-4 pounds over 12 weeks by eating half a grapefruit or drinking grapefruit juice with each meal and exercising regularly; many participants lost more than 10 pounds. It was hypothesized that the grapefruit reduced insulin levels, encouraging fat loss.

Things to do to Boost Your Metabolic Rate

Build Muscle Mass: Strength training builds lean muscle tissue, which burns more calories at work or at rest 24 hours a day, seven days a week. The more lean muscle you have, the faster your metabolism will be. How do you start strength training? Try some push ups, or a few squats or lunges. Use 5 lb free weights to perform simple biceps curls or triceps pulls.

Do not Skip Meals or drastically reduce your caloric intake, if you body senses that food is in short supply, it will slow your metabolism to conserve energy. Over time, the results are that when you do eat your body will be slower to use the calories as fuel, thus creating a backlog of unwanted pounds. Dive your meals into 6 different small meals/snacks through out the day.

Increase the amount of Protein in your Diet: Most researchers agree that protein helps to stabilize the secretion of insulin into your blood stream, a process that can affect metabolism. The average person would benefit from protein intake at a minimum of 70 grams or higher each day.

Increase movement: The more you move the more you burn. You can actually make a significant addition to the number of calories you burn each day by relatively minor changes in lifestyle; this can be as simple as taking the stairs instead of the elevator; park a distance from the mall or office, window shop with your friend rather than sit over coffee, walk the dog instead of just letting him out, clean house while you talk on the phone. Making these types of changes for just 20 minutes of your day will cause you to burn an additional 100 calories per day or an additional 1 or 2 pounds per month.

Walk: Go for an evening walk. Evening activity may be particularly beneficial. Many people's metabolism slows down toward the end of the day. Thirty minutes of aerobic activity before dinner increases your metabolic rate and may keep it elevated for another two or three hour. What that means for you: those dinner calories have less of a chance to take up permanent residence on your hips.

Weight Calendar

Sunday	Monday	Tuesday	Wednesday	Thursday	Friday	Saturday

Weight Calendar

Sunday	Monday	Tuesday	Wednesday	Thursday	Friday	Saturday

Weight Calendar

Sunday	Monday	Tuesday	Wednesday	Thursday	Friday	Saturday

Weight Calendar

Sunday	Monday	Tuesday	Wednesday	Thursday	Friday	Saturday

INDEX

A
Agave, 10

B
Benefits of ingredients, 8, 9

D
Drinks
  Apple milk shake, 55
  Lemonade, 52
  Strawberry, shake, 55
  Tea, cinnamon, 53
  Tea, Lemon, 53
  Yogurt, fruit, 54
  Yogurt, orange, 54

G
Grocery list, 6, 7

M
Metabolic Rate, boost, 61

O
Other Diets Defined, 59, 60

P
Planned meals, 12, 13, 14, 15, 16

S
Salad Recipes
  Beet & Yogurt, 31
  Cauliflower, 30
  Mediterranean, 33
  Pomegranate & Almond, 32
  Spinach, 36
  White Beans & Tuna, 35
  Vegetable & Fruit, 34
  Zucchini, 37

Sauces & Dressings, 38, 39

Soup Recipes
  Cabbage, 18
  Cabbage & Beets, 19
  Cabbage, Carrot, Pea, 25
  Chickpea, 26
  Broccoli, 22
  Fish, 23
  Spinach, 24
  Tomato, 20
  Vegetable, 21
  White Bean, 27
Soup, diet explained, 5

T
Tips, satisfy for sweets, 57

V
Vegetable Recipes
  Asparagus, almonds, 48
  Cauliflower, 42
  Carrots, sweet-sour, 49
  Green Beans, 44
  Mushrooms, 47
  Peppers with mushrooms, 46
  Spinach, chickpeas & Yogurt, 45
  Tomatoes, grilled, 43

W
Weight Calendar, 63

Made in the USA
Lexington, KY
02 March 2016